# Dr Dawn's Guide

Dr Dawn Harper is a GP based in Gloucestershire, working at an ....S surgery in Stroud. She has been working as a media doctor for nearly ten years. Dawn is best known as one of the presenters on Channel 4's award-winning programme *Embarrassing Bodies*, which has run for seven series and in 2014 celebrated its hundredth episode. Spin-offs have included *Embarrassing Fat Bodies* and *Embarrassing Teen Bodies*.

Dawn is one of the doctors on ITV1's *This Morning* and is the resident GP on the health show on LBC radio. She writes for a variety of publications, including *Healthspan* and *Healthy Food Guide*. Her first book, *Dr Dawn's Health Check*, was published by Mitchell Beazley. *Dr Dawn's Guide to Weight and Diabetes* is one of five Dr Dawn Guides published by Sheldon Press in 2015. Dawn qualified at London University in 1987. When not working, she is a keen horsewoman and an enthusiastic supporter of children's charities. Her website is at <www.drdawn.com>. Follow her on Twitter @drdawnharper.

# Overcoming Common Problems Series

*Selected titles*

A full list of titles is available from Sheldon Press,
36 Causton Street, London SW1P 4ST and on our website at
www.sheldonpress.co.uk

# Overcoming Common Problems Series

# Overcoming Common Problems Series

Overcoming Common Problems

# Dr Dawn's Guide to Weight and Diabetes

### DR DAWN HARPER

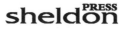

First published in Great Britain in 2015

Sheldon Press
36 Causton Street
London SW1P 4ST
www.sheldonpress.co.uk

The author and publisher have made every effort to ensure that the
external websites included in this book are correct and up to date at the
time of going to press. The author and publisher are not responsible for
the content, quality or continuing accessibility of the sites.

*British Library Cataloguing-in-Publication Data*
A catalogue record for this book is available from the British Library

ISBN 978-1-84709-356-1
eBook ISBN 978-1-84709-357-8

Typeset by Fakenham Prepress Solutions, Fakenham, Norfolk NR21 8NN
First printed in Great Britain by Ashford Colour Press
Subsequently digitally reprinted in Great Britain

eBook by Fakenham Prepress Solutions, Fakenham, Norfolk NR21 8NN

Produced on paper from sustainable forests

*Dedicated to my Mum and Dad
for their unwavering support*

# Contents

# Contents

# Introduction

When I was 12 years old, I was admitted to hospital with appendicitis. In those days, after the operation you stayed in hospital for a few days and, as I recuperated, I found I was fascinated with what the doctors and nurses were doing. By the time I was discharged, my decision was made – I wanted to be a doctor. Three years later, when careers advice was being handed out, I steadfastly refused to discuss anything else. I knew what I wanted to do and, like any self-respecting 15 year old, I knew much better than the adults around me! Finally, my headmistress called a meeting with my parents. She was concerned I was making a mistake. She told them I was a linguist, not a scientist, and that if, jointly, they could persuade me to rethink, I would have a very bright career ahead of me. Thank goodness they failed! I am lucky to love my job, all aspects of it, although I do have to concede that my teachers may have had a point as my working week today involves more time talking and writing about medical issues than it does actually practising them. In fact, when I wrote my first book in 2007, I dedicated it to my German teacher who I still see every year.

So what happened, and how did I get to where I am today? Well, fast forward a few years and I qualified in medicine at Charing Cross and Westminster Medical School. I still remember the day that I called home and simply said 'It's Dr Harper speaking'. I felt on top of the world. To this day every time I drive into London (which is very often!), I look right at the Charing Cross hospital in Fulham with fond memories. After I qualified I spent a number of years working in various medical specialties and took post-graduate exams to become a member of the Royal College of Physicians. I then spent some time working in Australia. They have a wonderful medical system, but it is not *free for all* as it is here in the UK, and, for the first time, I started to appreciate the real cost of treatment and just how wonderful our NHS is. I often say that the NHS is 'like your Mum' – she may not be perfect, but she has your best interests at heart and, one thing is for sure, you will miss her when she is gone. I hope that day never comes, but I do believe we all have a responsibility to look after her.

I have a responsibility as an individual, as a mother and as a doctor and broadcaster, to make sure that my family, my patients, my viewers and my readers are in the best position possible to understand any medical problems they have, and know what they can do to help themselves, which is one of the reasons I wanted to write this series of books – I hope you find them helpful.

For the last few years, I have been working as a doctor in the media alongside my clinical practice. I started by answering medical queries on a consumer health website, which lead to me being asked to write for various magazines and, ultimately, appear on television and radio. In 2013, we celebrated our one hundredth episode of *Embarrassing Bodies*. There have been several more episodes since, and I hope there will be more to come. I am now one of the regular doctors on ITV's *This Morning* and do a weekly Health Hour phone-in on LBC radio. My media work has shown me time and time again that people often leave the consulting room with unanswered questions. Maybe you forgot to ask, or maybe there simply wasn't enough time, and I guess that is the other reason for the Dr Dawn Guides. My aim for these books is to address all those unanswered questions.

This particular book is, perhaps, the most important. I have already alluded to the fact that there could come a time when we don't have an NHS as we know it, and actually that may not be down to politicians. It may be down to us, the public. We are already the fattest nation in Europe and, in the obesity stakes, are rapidly catching up with America. We have an obesity epidemic here in the UK and, if we don't reverse the trend, obesity alone could bankrupt our NHS. We live in an obesogenic society. Food is readily available and most of us are more sedentary in our day to day lives than our parents or grandparents were. It is just too easy to put on weight and, if everyone around us is overweight, it is also too easy to be lulled into a false sense of security that it is normal and nothing to worry about. I wish I could say obesity wasn't anything to worry about, but it is. In this book I will try to explain the health risks of carrying excess weight but also to help you make small changes that, literally, will make you look better, feel better and live longer.

Believe me, I know it's not easy. Every one of you picking up this book will have tried to lose weight in the past with varying degrees of success, but you are interested in this book because you have yo-yo'd back. You are not on your own – thousands of people before you have lost weight only to rebound back and, usually, with a few extra pounds to show for it. I am going to help you understand why you don't seem to be able to manage your weight long term, and will take you, step by step, through how you can take back the control you need to live a happier, healthier and even a longer life. In this book, I will show you how a few simple changes to your life could keep you feeling well and looking good for longer. Actually, no, for life! Eating well, exercising regularly and keeping stress under control will make you healthier, fitter and more confident. But don't panic, there is nothing in this book that will require superhuman will-power. In fact, the exact opposite is true. Most of us can stick to a restrictive diet for a week or two or cut out alcohol for short periods but very few can or even want to keep that up for months let alone for life. If lifestyle changes are to have any effect on health and longevity, they have to be achiev-able and sustainable, so I am not about to suggest that half the population train for a marathon. My aim in this book is simply to point you in the right direction to help you make very small changes to your lifestyle that you can stick to and that really give you the results you want. I know you can lose weight and keep it off for good, you just haven't been shown how to yet!

Before I start I'd like to take a quick look at how things have changed in recent decades. Heart disease is the biggest killer in the UK today. In fact, more than 600 people will die of the condition today, but why is heart disease now so prevalent a killer, when little over 150 years ago, along with cancer and dementia, it was extremely rare? Modern day Britain is obsessed with cleanliness and hygiene and thousands of column inches have been written about superbugs and flu pandemics but a comparison of Victorian and modern day life makes what we now think of as an infection- and disease-filled era, positively sparkle with good health. In Victorian Britain, 3 out of every 20 babies died before their first birthday and the average adult only lived into their forties. Infections such as cholera and typhoid sent many to an early grave, but women also died in childbirth, and many lives were lost in industrial accidents and domestic fires. Women used to cook on open fires and often their crinoline dresses caught fire while cooking. The Victorians did die young of heart failure not from clogged up arteries and morbid obesity, but due to infection from rheumatic fever – something that we rarely ever see in Britain today.

Few would disagree that we have come a long way in improving hygiene and infection control and, while some may find Health and Safety regulations restrictive, it is fair to say that a death in the workplace, or while cooking supper, is now so vanishingly rare that it would make headline news. Diabetes, heart disease and obesity seem to be the curse of modern day Britain. Cynics would argue that Victorians simply didn't live long enough to develop these conditions and, of course, that is partly true but I believe there is more to it than that. A quick look at the lifestyles and diets of Victorian Britain compared to today is revealing. In Victorian days you didn't drive your kids to school. There were no washing machines, vacuum cleaners or supermarket deliveries on the internet. The average adult used around 4000 calories a day simply doing the chores – they didn't need a gym membership or a personal trainer. Compare that to the average British adult today who uses little over half those calories daily, and the cause of the twenty-first century obesity epidemic starts to become obvious. If that's not frightening enough, compare your childhood to that of your children or grandchildren. I encourage my kids to get out and about as much as possible but, even so, they spend significantly more time in front of some form of screen than I ever did as a child. For the first time in over a century we are looking at a situation where our children may not outlive us – and it won't be cholera or typhoid that is to blame.

The Victorian diet was also very different. Victorians were more likely to be underweight than overweight. The reverse is true today, but many will be surprised to learn that despite being fat many of us are actually malnourished. We are getting enough (or in many cases too much) food but not enough nutrients. In Victorian times, there were no fast-food burger joints or pre-packaged foods. They had a low intake of salt, alcohol and tobacco. The 'five portions of fruit and veg a day' message hadn't been thought of but it didn't need to either – the average Victorian diet equalled more than ten portions a day. The diet was rich in whole grains, prebiotic fibre and omega-3 oils, which are so lacking today. In fact, our dietary intake of selenium, prebiotic fibre and sterols could be, on average, half what it was just 150 years ago. So what can we learn from the Victorians? Don't panic, I'm not about to suggest that we wash everything by hand and throw away all domestic appliances, but we do need to increase our exercise levels. With a little fine tuning we could significantly reduce the risks of those diseases that were virtually unheard of 150 years ago.

There is no doubt that we are all getting bigger. Our modern day lifestyles and easy access to plentiful food make it much harder for many of us to maintain a healthy body weight but, hopefully, I will help you make subtle changes to your life that will have a huge impact on your health and well-being.

# 1

# Am I overweight?

## Body mass index

There are a number of different ways of assessing weight. Perhaps the most common is the body mass index or BMI. Effectively, this is a measure of your weight in relation to your height. We would, after all, expect a tall person to weigh more than a short person. All doctors have BMI charts that tell them the healthy range of weight any individual should be for a given height. To calculate your BMI you simply need to know your weight in kilograms, and your height in metres (see Box). A healthy BMI is between 18.5 and 25 kilograms/m².

---

### How to calculate your BMI

Your BMI is your weight, measured in kilograms, divided by the square of your height, measured in metres.

$$BMI = weight \div height^2$$

You calculate the number for the square of your height by multiplying your height (in metres, remember) by itself.

$$BMI = weight \div (height \times height)$$

I weigh 52 kg and I am 1.63 m tall. So, for me, the calculation looks like:

$$BMI = 52 \div (1.63 \times 1.63) = 52 \div 2.66 = 19.57$$

My BMI is 19.57 kg/m², which means that I am currently a healthy weight.

---

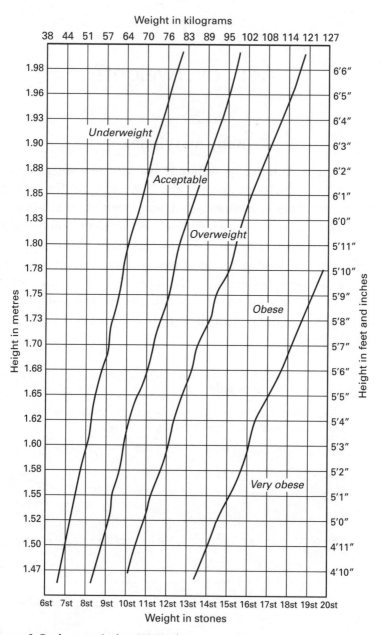

**Figure 1 Body mass index (BMI) chart**

*Source*: Taken from Dr Robert Povey, Dr Claire Hallas and Dr Rachel Povey, *Living with a Heart Bypass*, London, Sheldon Press, 2006, p. 82.

This calculation has nothing to do with fashion and dress size. It is a method of measuring a sensible, healthy weight for your height. I can afford to put on a few pounds before I would be classed as clinically overweight, but we all know how easy it is to put on a couple of kilos on a holiday or over the Christmas period. If we allow the extra weight to stay around, rather than getting ourselves back in check straight away, then it is easy for our BMIs to creep up. If I were to gain 14 kilos my BMI would be about to tip into the unhealthy range at 25, and if I allowed myself to put on another 13 kilos I would be classed as clinically obese. Take a look at the chart in Figure 1 to work out your BMI, or go to <www.nhs.uk/Tools/Pages/Healthyweightcalculator.aspx> to calculate it online.

But BMI has its failings. We know that muscle is more dense than fat, which is why, if you combine a weight loss programme with diet and exercise, you may notice your clothes feeling looser before the scales are registering much in the way of weight loss. Very fit, muscly athletes may have a BMI in the overweight, or sometimes even the clinically obese, range: fit rugby players, for example. Well-built, supremely fit, rugby players, because of the density of their muscle mass, may appear on paper to be of an unhealthy weight. They are, of course, at a very low risk of all the health complications associated with being overweight. BMI is a useful calculation for most of us, but there are other ways of assessing weight and there is an increasing move towards using waist circumference and hip to waist ratio rather than BMI alone.

## Waist circumference

Being overweight increases our risk of becoming type 2 diabetic, developing high blood pressure and heart disease, to name but a few of the health risks – more of that later. But it is not just how much we weigh that influences our risk; where we store that weight is also important. Weight stored on our thighs, bottom and hips is inactive – it contributes a little bit to our risk – but weight stored around our middles is more risky. I think of fat on our thighs as a storage barn full of fat waiting to be used in times of shortage, whereas fat around our middles is more like a factory full of fat – it is there in times of shortage, but it is also active and produces hormones and chemicals that increase our risk of developing weight-related health problems. So, if you took two identical women of identical height and weight, but one was an apple shape (storing weight round her middle) and the other a pear shape (storing weight around her hips), the apple-shaped woman would be more at risk of becoming diabetic or having high blood pressure than the pear. We can't help where we store our weight – that is genetically predetermined – but it does mean that people who store their weight around their middle have even more reason to keep their weight in check, and doctors are increasingly using waist circumference as an assessment of health risk.

Before we discuss the healthy measurements we should be aiming for, it is important that we know exactly how to measure our waists. It may sound daft, but, believe me, I have met far too many people happily wearing 34 inch waist trousers that were sitting snugly underneath a significantly larger waist! To measure your waist you need to feel for your hip bone and for the bottom of your ribs. The idea is to breathe out naturally (don't force your abdomen out, just gently exhale) and measure your circumference midway between these two points. It is always a good idea to check the measurement more than once to make sure that you have measured accurately. Women should have a waistline no greater than 80 cm, or 32 inches, and men no greater than 94 cm, or 37 inches (see Table 1). Waistlines greater than this are associated with significantly increased risks of high blood

**Table 1 Waist sizes linked to health risk**

| | Waist size | |
| --- | --- | --- |
| | Health at risk | Health at high risk |
| Men | Over 94 cm (37 inches) | Over 102 cm (40 inches) |
| Women | Over 80 cm (32 inches) | Over 88 cm (35 inches) |
| South Asian men | – | Over 90 cm (36 inches) |
| South Asian women | – | Over 80 cm (32 inches) |

Source: British Heart Foundation

pressure, heart disease and diabetes and, if you are of Asian descent, things get even tougher. Asian men, in particular, are at increased risk of these conditions, so the numbers are smaller – their waistlines should be no more than 90 cm (36 inches).

## Waist-to-hip ratio

We know that weight stored around our middles is more dangerous in terms of health risk, so a simple calculation of the ratio of your waist to hip measurements is another way of identifying if you are at risk. Measure your waist as I described in the previous section – at the midpoint between your hip bone and the bottom of your ribs. Your hip measurement should be taken at the widest point of your hips, and the ratio is simply calculated by dividing the waist number by the hip number. A ratio of 0.85 or more for women, or 1.0 or more in men, means you are carrying too much weight around your middle and it is time you addressed this before you run into trouble with your health.

## Percentage body fat

We need some fat to keep us insulated, to protect our organs, and as a source of stored energy but excess fat is bad for us and increases our risk of heart disease, diabetes and

**Table 2 Am I overweight?**

| Age range (years) | Body fat percentage | Weight classification |
|---|---|---|
| *Women* | | |
| 20–40 | <21 | Underweight |
| | 21–33 | Healthy |
| | 34–39 | Overweight |
| | >39 | Obese |
| 41–60 | <23 | Underweight |
| | 23–35 | Healthy |
| | 36–40 | Overweight |
| | >40 | Obese |
| 61–79 | <24 | Underweight |
| | 24–36 | Healthy |
| | 37–42 | Overweight |
| | >42 | Obese |
| *Men* | | |
| 20–40 | <8 | Underweight |
| | 8–19 | Healthy |
| | 20–25 | Overweight |
| | >25 | Obese |
| 41–60 | <11 | Underweight |
| | 11–22 | Healthy |
| | 23–27 | Overweight |
| | >27 | Obese |
| 61–79 | <13 | Underweight |
| | 13–25 | Healthy |
| | 26–30 | Overweight |
| | >30 | Obese |

high blood pressure. How much fat is allowed depends on your gender and your age. Some scales will calculate your percentage body fat for you, but you can work out your percentage body fat for yourself, using a simple calculation and an ordinary set of weighing scales and tape measure.

For women:  Body fat percentage = (1.20 × BMI)
+ (0.23 × Age) − 5.4

For men:  Body fat percentage = (1.20 × BMI)
+ (0.23 × Age) − 16.2

The guidelines in Table 2 will help you work out whether you have anything to worry about.

# 2

# Does being overweight matter?

As a doctor I have to say – yes! Being overweight does matter, and I think it matters on all sorts of levels. Of course it matters in terms of health risks, and in this chapter I will go into some of the diseases associated with carrying excess weight. Some of these diseases, such as diabetes and heart disease, will come as no surprise but others may not be quite so obvious, and they all represent good reasons for wanting to maintain a healthy weight.

But it's not just for health reasons that I think being overweight matters. I have met a few people over the years who seem genuinely content to be on the larger side, but I have met many more who struggle with their weight and feel miserable about it. As a GP, I think there are practical, emotional and physical reasons for keeping our weight in check. If you don't like your body, it is likely to mean that you have problems with self-confidence. At its worst, this can mean that you are less likely to have an active social life and it can also have a detrimental effect on your love life, with possible knock-on effects on your relationship as a whole. And there is no doubt that carrying extra weight leaves you feeling less energized.

We don't wake up one morning to discover that we are carrying a couple of extra stone that wasn't there the day before. If we did we would recognize very quickly how being overweight or obese leaves us feeling tired, more easily short of breath and more likely to have aches and pains. We gain weight very slowly. A couple of pounds here and there won't make any difference to how you feel day to day, but a couple of pounds added to a couple of pounds, and another couple of pounds, and it can soon take its toll. I often say to patients that if I were to set them off on their day with a rucksack carrying two or three stone of rocks, then at the end of the day they would feel shattered, their back would undoubtedly ache. They would probably have spent most of the day feeling hot, sweaty and breathless on fairly minimal exertion. Since nearly two-thirds of our adult population is overweight and a quarter of the adult population is clinically obese, this is exactly how these people feel every day. Maybe that is you and, because it has happened so gradually

**Table 3 Diseases that occur more frequently in the obese**

| Part of body | Disease |
| --- | --- |
| Head/brain | Cataracts |
| | Idiopathic intracranial hypertension |
| | Stroke |
| Heart | Angina |
| | Coronary heart disease |
| Lungs | Hypoventilation syndrome |
| | Obstructive sleep apnoea |
| | Pulmonary disease |
| Liver | Non-alcoholic fatty liver diseases |
| | Steatosis |
| | Steatohepatitis |
| | Cirrhosis |
| Gynaecological abnormalities | Abnormal menses |
| | Infertility |
| | Polycystic ovary syndrome |
| General | Cancer (breast, uterus, cervix, colon, oesophagus, pancreas, kidney, prostate) |
| | Diabetes |
| | Hypertension |
| | Osteoarthritis |
| | Severe pancreatitis |

over many months or years, this is normal for you and you have acclimatized. But you don't have to accept that – losing weight will leave you feeling more energized and in less pain. And, more than that, it will reduce your risks of developing a whole host of diseases (see Table 3).

## Diseases that are common in obese people

It will come as no surprise to you that heart disease, type 2 diabetes and high blood pressure are more common in the overweight and, of course, the more overweight you are the more at risk you are. However, many of my patients don't realize that some cancers, including breast cancer, colon cancer and ovarian cancer, are also more likely to strike the overweight. Being overweight means you are more likely to develop sleep apnoea which can leave you tired during the day and, undoubtedly, contributes to some road traffic accidents. And if you need surgery when you are overweight, virtually every possible post-operative complication, from infections to blood clots, is more likely to occur. Excess weight puts strain on your joints – particularly your back, hips, knees and feet – making osteoarthritis more common and joint replacement surgery less successful, because of the post-operative problems.

So whether it is diabetes or depression, the bigger you are the more likely you are to suffer. But it doesn't have to be all doom and gloom – the majority of these medical problems are reversible if you can get your weight back into a healthy range – you just need to be shown how, and you will, literally, feel like a new person!

# 3

# Why are we all overweight?

There is no doubt that we live in, what has been described as, an **obesogenic society** – food is readily available and most of us lead relatively sedentary lifestyles. Weight gain and loss is all about a very simple equation – if we put in more energy than we use up, we store the excess as fat. If we expend more than we take in, we will use up those stores and lose weight. So simple and easy in theory and yet incredible difficult to do in practice.

I often hear people complaining that it seems so much easier to gain weight than it is to lose it. The truth of the matter is that 3,500 calories equates to a pound of fat. If we consistently eat 500 calories a day more than we need, we will gain one pound in a week, four pounds in a month and almost a stone in three months. The problem is that it is so much easier to consistently eat 500 calories a day more than we need, but so much more difficult to stick to cutting back by 500 calories a day less than we need, which is why it can seem that weight goes on faster than it comes off! And, to be fair, some people seem to find it easier to keep their weight under control than others, so let's take a look at some of the factors influencing weight.

## Genetics

There has been a lot of talk about the genetics of obesity, and scientists have identified several genes that could be linked to a predisposition to gaining weight. I was tested for 12 of these genes for *Embarrassing Bodies*. As you can be either positive or negative for each of these genes, on average you would expect me to test positive for six but, in fact, I tested positive for eight! There is one particular gene, the *FTO* gene, which is sometimes referred to as the **fat gene**. As everyone has two copies of this gene, an individual can be fat/fat (has two copies of the fat gene), fat/thin (one copy of the fat gene and one thin gene) or thin/thin (two copies of the thin gene). I was surprised to learn that I am fat/fat which would suggest that I might gain weight easily. In fact, I am very careful about what I eat and exercise a great deal – often cycling up to 100 miles a week. My medical colleagues now tease me that when I stop this regime I am likely to really struggle with my weight. But my story is basically good news. We can't, as yet, do anything about the genes that we inherit, but they are not necessarily the curse that you may think and with some lifestyle changes we can override any pre-programming to weight gain that we have.

## Metabolism

It is a commonly held myth that bigger people have slower metabolisms. I often hear patients complain that they must have a slow metabolism because they really struggle with their weight; I can totally understand that logic, but in fact the exact opposite is true! Let's go back to that rucksack of rocks. If I was to put that on you today, you would have to use up more calories just breathing. Your basal metabolic rate, or BMR, is the number of calories you use simply to exist and breathe before you do any exercise. You can calculate your BMR using these formulas below. You will need to know your weight in kilograms, your height in centimetres and your age in years.

For women:  BMR = 65 + (9.6 × weight) + (1.8 × height) – (4.7 × age)

For men:  BMR = 66 + (13.7 × weight) + (5.0 × height) – (6.8 × age)

If you look at the equations closely, you will see that there is a direct link between weight and BMR – the heavier you are the higher your basal metabolic rate will be, not lower.

## Portion sizes

The odds are stacked against us here – whether it's a portion of chips or a bar of chocolate – the size of a standard portion has increased dramatically in recent years and so our idea of what is a reasonable amount of food to eat in one go has increased. We are surrounded by supersize everything, and there should, therefore, be no surprises that that predisposes us to being supersize people! Figure 2 overleaf gives you some idea of the portion sizes that you should be eating.

## Activity levels

I was once told, in a lecture on psychology, that people are like one of four animals – we are all, apparently, lions, elephants, dolphins or monkeys. The analogy was intended to describe personality traits: the lions are the leaders; the elephants are the solid, steadfast followers; the dolphins are the pleasers – they just want everyone to be happy – and the monkeys are the party people, who are on the go all the time. Look around at your friends and colleagues and you will identify lions, elephants, dolphins and monkeys among them. And I wouldn't mind betting that the monkeys are generally slimmer than the elephants! I am being over-simplistic, but people who fidget burn up significantly more calories than those that don't – fidgeting can account for as many as 500 calories a day!

*Grains*

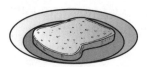

1 slice of bread

1 cup of rice, pasta
or cereal

*Fruit and vegetables*

1 portion of fruit or veg

½ cup of canned fruit

1 cup of salad or
cooked veg

*Dairy*

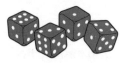
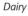

1 oz cheese

¾ cup of yogurt

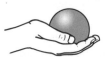

1 cup of milk

*Meat and alternatives*

3 oz meat, poultry or fish

2 small eggs or
1 large egg

2 tablespoons of peanut
butter

*Oils, spreads and dressings*

1 teaspoon of dressing,
oil, butter or cream
cheese (2 stacked 10 pence pieces
or top joint of thumb)

**Figure 2 Portion sizes**

## Eating habits

I remember being told as a child that you should eat breakfast like a king, lunch like a prince and supper like a pauper. Not only do very few of us do this, but also most of us probably don't even eat three meals a day. Lifestyles are increasingly busy and many of us will tend to snack while on the move rather than sit down to eat three square meals a day, and it is far too easy to underestimate your calorific intake if you are grazing throughout the day. Grazers are thought to underestimate their daily intake by anything from 500 to 1,000 calories a day.

# 4

# The benefits of weight loss

If you feel good about your body, the chances are you will feel better about yourself in general. You will feel more confident and have higher self-esteem, which translates into feeling more positive about life as a whole. You will feel more energized and, almost certainly, sexier, which will probably mean a happier sex life – and happier relationships too. But, as a doctor, it is the health benefits of maintaining a healthy weight that I think are most important.

If you are carrying a lot of excess weight the idea of getting down to a BMI of between 18.5 and 25 may seem totally daunting and unachievable and, while you may want to drop a few dress sizes for cosmetic reasons, it is important that you know that even modest weight loss will have profound effects on your health. If you are obese, losing just 10 per cent of your body weight will improve your health in many ways.

## Blood pressure

A healthy blood pressure should be lower than 140/90 mm Hg. The top number – 140 – is called the **systolic blood pressure**. This is the maximum blood pressure in your system caused by blood being pumped out of the heart by the muscular contraction of the heart wall. The lower number – 90 – is called the **diastolic blood pressure** and reflects the lowest pressure which occurs with the relaxation of the muscular heart wall. If your blood pressure is consistently greater than 160/90 mm Hg, your doctor will recommend medication. If it is between 140/90 mm Hg and 160/100 mm Hg, your doctor will probably talk to you about lifestyle changes in the first instance. That includes changes such as cutting down on salt intake, stopping smoking, increasing exercise and, yes, you guessed it . . . losing weight. But there is good news here. If an obese person loses just 10 per cent of their body weight, they can expect a fall of 10 mm Hg in both systolic and diastolic pressure, which can make the difference between needing to be on long-term medication and not!

## Impaired glucose tolerance

In non-diabetics, blood glucose (sugar) levels are regulated by a hormone released from the pancreas called **insulin**. Regardless of how much sugar you eat, in a normal healthy person, blood sugar levels are kept consistently within a narrow, normal range. Being clinically overweight or obese can mean that you become resistant to the effects of insulin such that your body struggles to maintain normal sugar levels. If blood tests show that your blood sugar levels are higher than they should be after drinking a fixed amount of glucose, but not high enough to be diagnostic of diabetes, then this is referred to as impaired glucose tolerance. If left unchecked this can progress to diabetes, but if an obese person loses just 10 per cent of their body weight this translates to at least a 30 per cent reduction in raised sugar levels, a 30 per cent improvement in sensitivity to insulin and a 40–60 per cent reduction in the rate of progression to diabetes.

## Diabetes

Being overweight massively increases your likelihood of developing type 2 diabetes, but if you are obese and you lose 10 per cent of your body weight, then abnormal fasting blood sugar levels fall in half of all cases. That could be the difference between needing prescription medication and not.

## Cholesterol

Not all cholesterol is bad – we have good cholesterol known as **high density lipoprotein** (HDL) and bad cholesterol, which is called **low density lipoprotein** (LDL). If you have heart disease or are diabetic, your doctor will want to reduce your total cholesterol but if not, your doctor will look at the ratio of total cholesterol to good (HDL) cholesterol and assess your risk from that; this risk assessment will take into account other risk factors such as blood pressure, age, gender and whether or not you smoke. If you have plenty of good (HDL) cholesterol you may not need treatment and, you've guessed it, if an obese person loses 10 per cent of their body weight then that has a significant impact on cholesterol and can cause a 10 per cent fall in total cholesterol.

So, even if you feel overwhelmed by the weight loss you want to achieve, focus on these things, and remember that even a relatively small loss of weight will make a huge difference to your health and well-being and, actually, to your longevity. Going back to that 10 per cent figure – if you are obese and you lose 10 per cent of your body weight, you are 40 per cent less likely to die as a result of your obesity. If that isn't motivation, I don't know what is!

# 5

# Is there a medical cause for my weight problem?

I am often asked this in surgery and sometimes the answer is 'Yes'. More frequently weight gain is a reflection of our lifestyle, but there are certain medications that can predispose to weight gain – I will list some of the more common culprits below – but don't ever be tempted to stop a prescription medication without first discussing it with your doctor, who will be able to talk you through any possible alternatives. The other thing to say is to be realistic about changes in weight and medication. Yes, all the medications listed below can be associated with weight gain, but if you have been on them for years and have only just started struggling with your weight, they are unlikely to be to blame. Most medicines that cause weight gain will do so as soon as you start taking them – so be honest with yourself.

## Medicines associated with weight gain

### Anti-depressants

Many anti-depressants, including tricyclics and selective serotonin reuptake inhibitors, can cause weight gain, although this can be a difficult one as depression can manifest itself as a loss of motivation meaning you are less active and therefore prone to weight gain.

### Contraceptives

Most hormonal contraceptives can lead to weight gain, but generally this is only of the order of a few pounds and should

occur soon after starting the medication. Both the combined pill and the mini pill can cause weight gain. The depo
injection can cause more significant weight gain and in my
experience it is often the women who were already carrying
a little extra weight who struggle the most. If you are putting
on a lot of weight on hormonal contraception, you need to
talk to your doctor, even if it is probably not related to the
pill itself, as, if you are clinically obese, you could be at risk
of deep vein thrombosis; overweight women taking the mini
pill may need a different dose.

## Hormone replacement therapy

Concern over weight gain is one of the most common reasons
women give me for not wanting to start hormone replacement therapy (HRT) and, to be fair, it can cause a small gain
in weight. Interestingly though, the menopause is a time of
change and that includes for your metabolism, which is why
so many women put on a few pounds in their 50s. We used
to talk a lot about middle-aged spread. We are now more
politically correct and it's a term that we rarely hear, but that
doesn't mean it doesn't happen! I have met lots of women in
my time who have declined HRT on the grounds of worries
over weight gain only to return a few months later (and a
few pounds heavier). The weight gain is down to changes in
our metabolism as we go through the change, but of course
if it starts when we start HRT, then the HRT gets the blame!

## Steroids

Taking steroids for a long time undoubtedly cause weight
gain, typically around the midriff, but if you are on steroids long term you absolutely mustn't stop them abruptly.
This can be very dangerous, so speak to your doctor about
whether you would be able to wean down.

## Diabetic medication

Some anti-diabetic tablets and insulin can cause weight gain, which, of course, is not ideal as carrying extra weight is in itself a cause of type 2 diabetes. There is one anti-diabetic medication, **metformin**, which has the opposite effect and can help with weight control, so have a chat with your doctor.

## Epilepsy medication

Some anti-convulsants are prone to cause weight gain, but again to stop these medications without talking to your doctor is very risky so please don't be tempted to take things into your own hands.

## Beta blockers

These drugs have a number of uses. You could be on them to protect your heart or to control blood pressure. They are also used for anxiety and to prevent migraine. Whatever their role they can cause weight gain – so if you are concerned have a chat with your doctor about possible alternatives.

## Anti-psychotic medication

Most anti-psychotics can be associated with weight gain but stopping these without medical supervision can be harmful so always check with your doctor first.

## Medical conditions associated with weight gain

Probably the best known condition associated with weight gain is an underactive thyroid. It can be tested for with a simple blood test and, certainly, if your weight gain is associated with an intolerance of the cold, fatigue, dry skin and hair, and a tendency to constipation, it should be checked out.

Women with polycystic ovary syndrome are prone to weight gain too and find it more difficult to lose weight than most of us, which is doubly tough, because losing weight helps alleviate the symptoms of the condition, such as acne, unwanted facial hair, period problems and difficulties with fertility.

Any condition that causes fluid retention will also show on the scales, although the weight is fluid not fat; this includes having a weak heart or problems with your liver or kidneys.

# 6

# Why can't I keep my weight under control?

I have lost count of the number of people I have met over the years who tell me how they have managed to lose weight in the past, often several stone, but then put it back on and, sadly more often than not, put it all back on and some more. This yo-yo dieting is extremely common, and really not good for your self-esteem as much as anything else. So let's take a look at some of the common pitfalls when it comes to getting your weight under control.

## Unrealistic expectations

We are constantly bombarded with celebrity-endorsed diets that promise you will drop a dress size in a week. We live in a quick fix culture – and who wouldn't want to achieve their ideal weight loss in as short a period of time as possible? Unfortunately, the truth is that weight lost slowly – one to two pounds a week – is far more likely to stay off. It takes time, and involves making long-term sustainable changes, but it gets the results you want. So be realistic with yourself – if you have just been invited to the party of the year in a fortnight's time and need to lose the best part of a stone to fit into that little black dress, then harness that emotion as a trigger for change – but choose a different outfit and save the little black dress for a couple of months time when you will have lost the weight and feel like a million dollars!

## Denial of current eating habits

I will talk about food diaries in more depth later but if you are overweight, the simple truth is that you are eating too much for your current activity level and it is incredibly easy to kid ourselves about the amount we eat. People often tell me they are not big eaters. They are not intentionally lying to me or themselves. They genuinely believe they are not and that they are cursed by a sluggish metabolism that means they are prone to weight gain. We all do it to a degree. If asked what we have eaten during the course of a day, we are likely to describe our meals and may well forget all about any snacks or drinks between meals. Milky drinks and many soft drinks are laden with calories, which soon add up to explain a big daily calorie count. And it is a well recognized fact that people who graze and pick at food throughout the day are likely to underestimate their daily calorie intake by anything between 500 and 1,000 calories a day! If you are going to achieve long-term weight loss, then dealing with snacking and grazing is going to have to be high on your agenda.

## Overly restrictive diet regimes

Many fad diets require you to exclude certain food groups or always combine certain foods. Anyone can cut out some-thing they like, or stick to a very strict regime, for a short period of time but the fact is that at some point you will falter and unless you have dealt with your relationship with food and made changes that you can stick with for life, then you are setting yourself up to fail. It is almost impossible to stick to very restricted diets and maintain any kind of normal social life, which means you either fall off the social radar while you try to maintain such a restrictive regime or you put yourself in temptation's way. Neither option is going to be good for your self-esteem. Setting yourself up for a fall is bound to leave you feeling guilty, and cutting yourself off from friends and family will make you miserable, which in turn could lead to a binge of comfort eating.

## The 'all or nothing' philosophy

Human nature means that we will occasionally let ourselves down. Whether it is dieting, training or studying, you will have days when your willpower and drive let you down. That's a fact. Don't beat yourself up about it. It just shows you are human, but too many of us make one mistake and give up altogether. It is important to recognize this – one day of bingeing in the biscuit tin doesn't have to mean you spiral out of control, but in the past that one day may have heralded the end of *whatever* diet you were on and the beginning of the yo-yo back to being overweight. If this is you, you need to recognize that and when the let-down day happens, don't fall apart! Dust yourself off, and get back on the wagon. A pound of fat is equivalent to 3,500 calories, so let's assume you have had a really bad day when you just let yourself go and munched your way through an extra 3,500 calories. That just means you will have put on a pound in weight and if you get yourself back in line the next day, you will soon be back on target. But, if you then allow yourself to do the same thing every day for the next week, because you have fallen victim to the 'all or nothing' philosophy, then it is easy to see how that unintentional weight gain could be half a stone. Remember this when you have a bad day, because you *will* have a bad day. The important thing is not to allow one bad day to lead to another and another. Put it behind you and move forward.

## Denial of current exercise habits

A bit like eating habits where we kid ourselves that we eat much less than we actually do, many of us overestimate just how much exercise we do. When I ask patients about exercise I am often told 'I'm on my feet all day with three kids' or 'I never stop at work'. Of course, anything we do to keep us mobile is good, but when I talk about exercise, I mean doing something that makes you huff and puff every day. Just 30 minutes is enough, but you need to be puffing. If you are gasping for breath, you are overdoing it but if you can chat quite happily without feeling short of breath you need to push yourself harder. And, of course, how easily you get to the puffing stage will depend on how active or inactive you have been. If you are carrying a lot of extra weight and have let formal exercise slip from your daily routine for a long while, then maybe keeping small children occupied and active *will* make you puff. But if you have an office-based job, it can be very difficult to achieve the recommended 10,000 steps a day. However, if you set your mind to it you will be amazed at how quickly your fitness will improve, and the knock-on effects are that you will feel more energized and your sleep will improve, meaning you face each new day with a fully recharged battery ready to face whatever challenges are presented to you.

## The wrong time

We often talk about setting a quit date when we talk to people about giving up smoking and, in just the same way, it is important that you are in the right frame of mind to make changes to your life and address your weight. I sometimes meet people, who for whatever reason have decided they will tackle smoking, weight and alcohol all at the same time. It seems logical in some ways that if you are looking for a healthy lifestyle you address all your issues, but there are potential pitfalls here. Don't be too hard on yourself – if you set the bar too high then it is going to be very hard to stick to and you could easily find yourself in that 'all or nothing' territory where one sneaky cigarette means you just give up on the whole new regime. You know yourself better than anyone and for some people dealing with everything all at once is the right thing, but that doesn't mean it is right for everyone and some of us find change easier to achieve in manageable stages. If this is you, deal with your most urgent problem first and make sure you are on track with that before moving up a level.

Spend some time thinking about the points I have raised here. Knowing your limitations and understanding why you have had problems in the past is part way to succeeding in the future. Weight loss isn't easy – if it were, we would all have BMIs in the healthy range, and there would be no need for a book like this. Losing weight is hard. It takes a lot of effort and focus, so make sure you are in the best place to set off on your new journey. Understanding your weaknesses and preparing for how you will cope with your bad days will help you keep on track.

# 7

# Getting started

You may be champing at the bit to get started and, if you are really ready, that's fine – but, to give yourself the best chance to succeed this time, you may need to spend some more time identifying your weaknesses. We all have them and there is nothing wrong with that; we just need to know how to deal with them. I am lucky in many ways. I don't have a sweet tooth so I can live with chocolate and biscuits in the cupboard for weeks without being tempted to eat them. That's not because I have more willpower than you. It is just because they don't appeal. But pass me a plate of cheese and then I struggle not to eat it all. It took me a long while to recognize this in myself but, now that I know, I try to avoid buying cheese for a while when I am trying to get myself back in check; for example, after a holiday or the Christmas break when most of us overindulge.

Your weaknesses may be glaringly obvious to you, but they may not be. It really is worth spending a couple of weeks before you start your new healthy living regime just documenting what you eat, when and why. And I mean everything. So if it is polishing off the spare chips from the kids' plates as you were clearing the table, you need to write it down – and try to think about why you ate them. Was it because you were hungry and the temptation was just too much? Was it just because they were there and you had eaten them before you even really had time to think about it? This is important because the most difficult part of your diet will be not cheating.

We all lead busy lives and it is amazing how easy it is to overeat, especially snacks. If you are really honest with yourself during your two-week diary keeping stage, you will very quickly be able to see your weak points. It is hard, I know, because as soon as you start to document things, it is human nature to start to alter what you do because, by definition, you are thinking about it. Try hard not to, and when you are at the end of your fortnight you will have a very clear record of your eating habits. There will be things that you knew all along, but other parts will surprise you. If you go for second helpings, try to make a note of how long you left it before you were reaching for the serving spoon and note whether you were having more because you were still feeling hungry – or because it was just so tasty.

So, now you have the facts in front of you and have identified your weaknesses, we are almost ready to get started. Whatever your weak points are, we need to make a plan as to how we deal with them. So let's just say it is chocolate biscuits. First of all ask yourself if you really need them in the house? Why do you buy the biscuits? Are they just too irresistible when you are doing the shopping? Can you force yourself not to go down that aisle? Are there times when you feel stronger than others? Could you time your weekly shop to be done when your willpower seems to be stronger? Have you considered internet shopping? Of course, if you live with other people who eat them then it is unfair to ask them to go without unless they are really behind you on this new journey and are happy to do so. If you have to have them in the house, are there some types of chocolate biscuits which are less tempting than others? Could you substitute those? If you really have to have chocolate biscuits in the house, try leaving yourself a note on the biscuit tin. Nothing nasty but maybe something along the lines of 'Do you really want this? If you do, you can have one if you still feel the same way in 5 minutes'. You would be amazed how often you will find your willpower in just a few minutes.

I had one lovely patient on *Embarrassing Fat Bodies* who had worked incredibly hard and lost 8 stone. She had so much to be proud of. She did it on her own with a healthy-eating and regular-exercise plan. It took her months but, believe me, she was unrecognizable physically and emotionally. Her lightbulb moment had been collecting a set of holiday snaps from the chemist. The first photograph was one of her sitting on a boat in the Mediterranean. She was a big girl, and she said that when she saw that photograph she saw herself as others saw her and she became very upset. We have long accepted that anorexics see a different image in the mirror than we do – they see fat bits that simply aren't there – and I believe this lady saw a different image in the mirror. She knew she was buying size 26 clothes, but in her mind she had kidded herself that she was a size 18 and she was comfortable with that. That photograph forced her to take her head out of the sand and accept that she was unhealthily overweight. She hated that picture – but she used it to her advantage. She kept it in the front of her purse so that every time she thought she wanted a burger, or a binge on chocolate, she had to get past that photograph to get to her money and nine times out of ten that image was enough to help her decide against her moment of weakness. She had a strategy that worked for her, and kept her on track most of the time. Your strategy may be something totally different but, with a bit of thought, you will be able to formulate a plan that will help you in moments of weakness.

# 8

# Healthy eating

The whole ethos of this book is about making small but sustainable changes – so don't panic. I have always been a firm believer that there is no such thing as a bad food, just plenty of bad diets. There is nothing wrong with chocolate or crisps as treats, but incorporate them into your diet every day and you are likely to run into trouble! When my children were small I used to have what I called the treats cupboard, where I kept biscuits and cake. As they got older and could open the cupboard and help themselves, we laughed that if a treat was a treat, it had to be just that – something special that you indulge in occasionally and not part of everyday life!

In the modern, western world we have rather lost sight of what is a healthy balanced diet. We live in an obesogenic society where food (and often the wrong food) is plentiful and we are all more sedentary than we were. I know my children spend more time sitting in front of some sort of screen than I ever did. They are active kids, but with the availability of laptops, tablets, games consoles and 24-hour television, it is so easy to spend much of our waking day sitting down. In a nutshell, what that means is that if we don't make conscious decisions to deal with our lifestyles we are going to be fighting an uphill battle with our weight.

So what is healthy eating? Well I'll tell you what it is not – cutting out whole food groups or only eating food of a certain colour. It is about getting the right balance of all the food groups and in the right proportions. The UK government have designed the **Eatwell plate** (see Figure 3 overleaf) to demonstrate what a healthy diet should look like.

**Fruit and vegetables 33%**

**Bread, rice, potatoes, pasta 33%** and other starchy foods

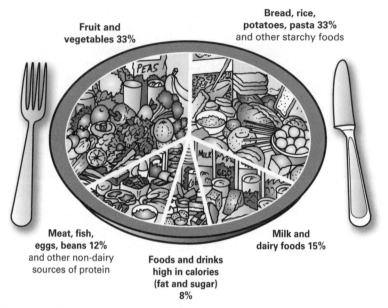

**Meat, fish, eggs, beans 12%** and other non-dairy sources of protein

**Foods and drinks high in calories (fat and sugar) 8%**

**Milk and dairy foods 15%**

**Figure 3  The Eatwell plate**

*Source*: Adapted from the diagram at <www.dh.gov.uk/health/2012/06/about-the-eatwell-plate>.

## Starchy foods

Starchy foods contain carbohydrate, which is an essential source of energy in our diet. Many diets recommend cutting out carbohydrates or keeping your intake to a minimum. We are back to the *no such thing as a bad food, just a bad diet* argument here. Carbohydrates are not bad for you but, if eaten in excess, the body will lay down the extra calories as fat stores for leaner times and to be honest it's not so much the food itself as the way it is cooked. Let's look at potatoes – a great source of starch but if you deep fry them in fat then you are loading on the calories. Starchy foods include bread, potatoes, pasta and rice and, as a general rule, wholegrain varieties are better than the types made from refined grains. At least half of the grains you eat should be whole grains and, to be honest, the greater the proportion the better. Wholegrain simply means that the bran hasn't been removed from the grain by milling, so they are higher in fibre; wholegrain foods include brown rice, brown pasta and brown bread. Refined grains have been milled, which strips out the bran, and foods made from refined grains include white bread, white rice and white pasta. It can be difficult to tell though as some 'brown bread' may be brown because it has added food colouring, so get into the habit of looking at food labels for the word *whole*.

## Fruit and vegetables

It's good to know that the five portions of fruit and vegetables message is getting out there. There has been much debate about whether this recommendation should be increased but, for me, if I could ensure that we all achieved our *five a day*, then I think we would be getting somewhere! Many people don't realize that frozen, canned and dried fruit and vegetables all count. Actually, fresh fruit juice also counts but only as one portion, irrespective of how much you drink, and that is because much of the fibre is removed during the process of juicing; the importance of fruit and vegetables in your diet is because they contain vitamins, minerals and some carbohydrate, mainly in the form of sugar, but also fibre. I will discuss what constitutes a portion in a later section.

## Meat, fish and other protein

Protein is an essential part of our diet. We need it to repair tissues and build muscle. Protein-rich foods are also a good source of vitamin B12, which is vital to maintain a healthy nervous system and make new red blood cells. They also tend to be a good source of iron, zinc and magnesium. We should all be eating at least two portions of oily fish a week as it is rich in omega-3 oils, which help prevent against heart disease and keep our skin and bones healthy. Oily fish include mackerel, sardines, trout and salmon.

## Milk and dairy

These foods are rich in calcium, which is essential for bone health. They also provide protein and B vitamins.

## Fat

Fat is the most energy-dense food, which is why a high-fat diet will predispose to weight gain. Most of us probably eat too much saturated fat, which is the fat found in butter, cheese, pastries, cakes and biscuits. Saturated fats and trans fats can raise cholesterol levels and increase the risk of heart disease so your fat intake should be no more than a third of your total calorie intake and, of this, only a third should be saturated or trans fats. It's a case of getting into the habit of checking food labels. This will seem very time consuming at first, but you will be amazed at how quickly you get used to knowing what you are looking for. Simple things like swapping butter for olive oil (rich in unsaturated fat) will make a significant difference to your health.

## Sugar

Most of us eat too much sugar and when you start analysing your diet you may be shocked at just how much sugar you are consuming. Beware 'low-fat' foods. Very often the fat is substituted with sugar to enhance the flavour, so you may think you have been choosing healthy options only to find that your sugar intake is too high. Most soft drinks are also laden with sugar – you would be surprised by how much you can reduce your daily calorific intake simply by swapping canned drinks for water.

## Salt

We have got used to a high-salt diet. Too much salt increases the risk of developing high blood pressure, which in turn increases the risk of heart attacks and strokes. We really should limit our daily intake to 6 grams and, when you start looking at the hidden salt in processed foods, you will be shocked by the amounts. Try to keep the amount of processed foods you eat to a minimum and, when cooking from scratch, limit the amount of added salt. At first food will taste bland but human taste buds adapt very quickly and, within a couple of weeks, you will wonder how you managed to eat such salty food!

## Alcohol

I guess I shouldn't be including alcohol in a chapter about a healthy, well-balanced diet but I promised you this book would be realistic and most of us do enjoy a drink. As I have said before, there is no such thing as a bad food (or in this case drink) – it is all about moderation. Recommended limits for alcohol are just 14 units a week for women and 21 for men and, I'm afraid I am going to frighten you now, that is significantly less than you think. We used to refer to a unit as a small glass of wine, half a pint of beer or a single measure of spirit but as beers and wines have become stronger we need to rethink this. The simple way to calculate your alcohol intake is by looking at the percentage alcohol in the drink you are drinking. The percentage alcohol shows you the number of units in a litre of that drink; so, for wine, a 75 cl bottle is three-quarters of a litre (75 cl = 750 ml; 1 litre = 1000 ml), so if the wine contains 12 per cent alcohol, the number of units in the bottle is three-quarters of 12 = 9 units. If you are pouring a glass at home it is likely to be a 250 ml glass and that will contain three units not one. So beware of alcohol. It is laden with hidden calories and will play havoc with your willpower!

## Calorie comparisons

As a rough guide, carbohydrates and proteins contain about 4 calories per gram, alcohol contains 7 calories per gram and fat contains 9 calories per gram.

### What is a portion?

Portion size is probably one of the biggest problems in the western diet. We have simply got used to overeating. You only have to look at the size of a Mars Bar – I am sure they have doubled in size since I was a kid and, of course, what that says to us, in a subliminal way, is that that large bar of chocolate is a totally appropriate amount to eat in one go on your own. It's not!

The best way to regulate your portions is to invest in scales, jugs and spoons, and smaller plates, bowls and wine glasses as we know that people eat up to as much as 50 per cent more from larger plates; sticking to smaller wine glasses will help you regulate your alcohol intake. But you are not going to be able to carry your dieting equipment with you wherever you go! If you get into the habit of measuring food at home though, you will soon learn to recognize what size a portion should be, and if you don't have your measuring devices to hand, here is a rough guide to what size portions you should eat:

- your palm is the size of a portion of meat or fish (approximately 150 grams);
- your cupped hand is the size of a portion of pasta or rice (about half a cup);
- both cupped hands is the size of a portion of salad (about one cup);
- your index finger is the size of a portion of cheese (about one tablespoon);
- your thumb is the size of a portion of jam (about one teaspoon).

## Dr Dawn's traffic light foods

As I have said before there is no such thing as a bad food but I like to group foods using the *traffic light* system.

- *Red foods* These are foods you need to be wary of. They

are the treats. Eat too many and you will really struggle to keep your weight under control. I guess there will be no surprises in this group – biscuits, chocolate, cake, crisps and alcohol all feature on my red list but that doesn't mean you can't have them. The minute you deny yourself for ever something you enjoy, you will become fixated on it – and it is only a matter of time before you cave in. So don't go there. If you love crisps you can tell yourself until you are blue in the face that you will never touch a crisp again but, as sure as night follows day, we both know that at some point you will waver. So be realistic. Red foods are for high days and holidays. Enjoy them occasionally, but don't let yourself indulge on a daily basis.

- *Amber foods* These are nutritious foods that should be incorporated in a well-balanced diet, but be careful about portion size as it is easy to clock up some serious calories if you are eating too much. In this group I include meat, fish, seafood, eggs, cereals, butter, dairy products and condiments such as chutney and mayonnaise.
- *Green foods* These are the low calorie foods. Fruits and vegetables are in this group. Just enjoy! Yes, many fruits are high in natural sugars, but these are so much better for you than the refined sugars in biscuits and cakes so get into the habit of swapping any snacks from red foods to green ones.

If you're not sure how many calories the foods you are eating have, this information is readily available on websites such as <www.weightlossresources.co.uk>, or apps such as *MyFitnessPal*, <www.myfitnesspal.com>. Table 4 overleaf suggests some ways you could cut your consumption of saturated fat. The cooking method makes a big difference to levels of fat. It's better to grill, steam or oven bake food instead of frying. If you must fry something, cook using a small amount of olive oil at a low temperature. You could also try sautéing in a little water or tomato juice.

**Table 4 Foods high in saturated fat and the low-fat alternative**

| | Avoid | Low-fat alternative |
|---|---|---|
| Snacks | Crisps/savoury snacks cooked in oil | Fresh or dried fruit, handful of nuts |
| Fats for cooking and spreading | Lard, dripping, ghee, cream and butter | Olive, sunflower, soya or rapeseed (blended vegetable) oils, margarines and spreads; store oils in a sealed container in a cool, dark place to prevent rancidity |
| Meat | Fatty products (sausages, burgers, pâté, salami, meat pies and pasties) | Lean cuts of meat and mince (check labels or ask the butcher); trim off fat<br>Skinless chicken and turkey<br>Vegetarian options (e.g. lentils, chickpeas and soya) |
| Fish | Deep fried (e.g. takeaway) fish and chips | Oily fish such as salmon, mackerel and sardines |
| Sauces | Creamy or cheesy sauces | Tomato or vegetable-based sauces |
| Dairy | Full-fat varieties | Skimmed (or at least semi-skimmed) milk, reduced-fat cheddar and low-fat yoghurt<br>Try grating cheese or using a strongly flavoured variety, which may mean you need to use less Edam, Camembert, Brie, reduced fat cheddar and cottage cheese contain less fat than many full-fat hard cheeses such as standard cheddar, Stilton, Parmesan and cream cheese |

*Source*: Adapted from British Dietetic Association

# What about second helpings?

There is nothing wrong with second helpings if you really need them, but try this little experiment. Put all the food you are going to eat in a single meal on your table and sit down to eat. Actually promising yourself that you will only eat sitting down is a good habit to get into. It means you are less likely to graze on canapés, nuts and crisps. You won't clear the kids' plates of leftover chips on your way to the sink, and you won't be able to cheat on portion size. You are also likely to eat more slowly, giving your brain a chance to register that your stomach is full. If when you have finished your plate and you still want more, promise yourself you can have it if you still want it in 15 minutes. It can take a while for the hormones released from our gut to tell our brains that we are full so give them a chance and, more often than not, you will start to feel full and decide against that second helping.

### Dr Dawn's top ten tips for slimmer eating

1  Identify your weaknesses.
2  Don't buy foods that will lead you astray.
3  Buy smaller plates, bowl and glasses.
4  Put all your food on your plate before you start eating.
5  Reduce your portion size by a third.
6  Sit down to eat.
7  Eat slowly.
8  Only go back for second helpings if you have allowed your first serving to digest for 15 minutes.
9  Keep healthy snacks with you to combat hunger pangs.
10  Drink more water.

# 9

# What about exercise?

There is no doubt that the best way to lose weight, and keep it off, is to combine a healthy-eating programme with regular exercise – but you need to pick your exercise. Many gym memberships are paid by well-intentioned people who part with their hard-earned cash, but give up going after a few weeks. Just paying your monthly subscription isn't going to be enough, you have to go – and go regularly! So now is another time to have a think and be honest with yourself. If you hate the gym, it doesn't matter how smart the facilities look or how many of your friends are raving about the place, you may force yourself to stick with it for a few weeks, maybe even a few months, but, as sure as eggs are eggs, you won't be going this time next year. And exercise is like healthy eating. You need to make small changes that, hand on heart, you think you will be able to keep up for good. I know this because, over the years, I have joined gyms. I join in January and, by Spring, I have usually fallen by the wayside – and that's because I get bored in a gym.

A few years ago I was run over by a car and shattered my left knee. Part of my rehabilitation involved sitting on a static bicycle in a physiotherapy gym, trying to flex my knee enough to do a single revolution. When I achieved this, I was so desperate to build the strength up in my damaged leg and regain full mobility, that I started cycling in the lanes near my house. I found that this was something I really enjoyed. Ten minutes on a bike in the gym and I'm clock watching but cycling in the countryside just ticked boxes for me, and I started cycling with friends in the village. I have always been a great believer in exercising with friends because when your motivation is low, they will spur you on and you will do the same for them. Before I knew it, I had signed up for a charity ride from London to Paris – and that ticked another box. There is nothing like the fear of failure to make sure you get out and train whatever your mood or the weather outside. So, I learned a lot about myself: I prefer exercising outside: I need friends to force me out when I'm feeling lazy; and I need a challenge to make me stick to my training schedule. The boxes you need to tick may be completely different and may not be obvious to begin with, but as you start your new healthy living regime, it is worth giving this some thought. Maybe you love dancing? A dance class is a great way to exercise. Perhaps you could help a friend walk their dog? Maybe it could be something as simple as walking with a work colleague at lunchtimes?

## Keeping active and exercising regularly

Anything we can do to keep moving will burn calories. We recommend that everyone walks at least 10,000 paces a day and, ideally, that should be your baseline on top of which you do your formal exercise but – again – don't be unrealistic about your goals. If you have been something of a couch potato in recent years, then just achieving 10,000 steps a day will be a major achievement. And it can be surprisingly difficult to do. The average pace is 50–75 cm long which means that 10,000 steps is walking 5–7.5 km in a day just going about your business! A while back I decided to practise what I preach and invested in a pedometer. I think of myself as quite an active person and certainly at weekends I had no problem clocking up my 10,000 paces. Busy days in surgery were a totally different matter, and I found that sitting at my desk calling in patients meant it was easy to get to 6.30 pm and be frighteningly short of my target. Then, I decided to get up and walk to the waiting room rather than use the intercom calling system. It meant I could maintain my activity levels on my surgery days and I actually prefer it. It is so much more personal than calling people through with the intercom. This simple change meant that I was staying on target and, in this day of internet technology, emails, texts and all the other ways of communicating with the outside world without actually moving, it can be all too easy to get to the end of your working day without having moved much at all.

It doesn't matter what you do, but if your job is sedentary you will have to make a definite decision to move more. Maybe get off the bus or the tube a stop early? Maybe use the stairs instead of an escalator or a lift? Maybe promise yourself that you will walk over to your colleague's desk to discuss an issue, rather than just press 'send' on an email? Whatever you decide to do, invest in a pedometer and start counting your daily steps. This is what I call baseline activity. Once you have achieved this, we need to think about exercise on top and, ideally, you should be aiming for 30 minutes a day. It doesn't matter what it is, but you need to get a bit short of breath doing it. The sort of shortness of breath that means you can only talk in short phrases and need to catch your breath. If you are gasping for air you are overdoing it and need to take the pressure off, but if you are chatting happily then don't kid yourself – you may be keeping active but you are not truly exercising and you need to push yourself a bit harder!

If you want to get a little more technical, buy yourself a heart rate monitor to wear while you are exercising. When you are fit, you should aim for a pulse rate between 70 and

85 per cent of your maximum heart rate (MHR). If you are just starting out, 60 per cent of your MHR is probably more realistic. You can calculate your MHR by subtracting your age from 220 if you are a man, or 210 if you are a woman. So, if you are a man aged 40, your MHR is:

220 − 40 = 180.

Your optimum training range is 70–85 per cent of 180, which is:

70% of 180 = (70 ÷ 100) × 180 = 126 beats per minute.

85% of 180 = (85 ÷ 100) × 180 = 153 beats per minute.

The great thing about exercise is that it burns calories (see Table 5) – but it also does so much more. If you exercise vigorously, you will boost your metabolism for the next 36 hours. What this means, in real terms, is that you will burn more calories just sitting at your desk than an identical person who hadn't done the exercise.

Table 5 How many calories will I burn?

| Activity | 9 stone | 11 stone | 14 stone |
|---|---|---|---|
| Aerobics – low impact | 295 | 352 | 431 |
| Aerobics – high impact | 413 | 493 | 604 |
| Lifecycle – light effort | 325 | 387 | 474 |
| Lifecycle – moderate effort | 413 | 493 | 604 |
| Lifecycle – vigorous effort | 620 | 739 | 906 |
| Running – 12 min/mile | 472 | 563 | 690 |
| Running – 8.6 min/mile | 679 | 509 | 992 |
| Running – 6 min/mile | 944 | 1126 | 1380 |
| Strength training | 472 | 563 | 690 |
| Swimming, vigorous | 590 | 704 | 863 |
| Swimming, backstroke | 472 | 563 | 690 |
| Swimming, breaststroke | 590 | 704 | 863 |
| Swimming, butterfly | 649 | 774 | 949 |
| Swimming, leisurely | 354 | 422 | 518 |
| Walking – moderate pace | 207 | 246 | 302 |
| Walking – very brisk pace | 236 | 281 | 345 |

Figures give the average number of calories burned per hour for each exercise for people of different weights.

# 10

# Can my doctor help?

As a GP I am very concerned about the obesity epidemic. So much so, that I fear for the future of the NHS. I have seen the numbers of diagnoses of type 2 diabetes rocket in recent years and experts are predicting that, if we don't do something to stop this trend, as many as one in three adults could have type 2 diabetes by 2050. We simply can't afford that, so we all have to do what we can to help overweight people to control their weight in a society which seems to conspire against maintaining a healthy BMI.

Your doctor has a number of different ways to help you. To start with, your doctor will be able to tell you whether you have any of the conditions linked to obesity – this on it's own works as a great motivator for some. Simply weighing you at regular intervals, so that you feel accountable for your weight, will help and many practices have the facility to prescribe exercise, which is a huge help if you know you work well in a class environment but don't have the cash to spend on these things. Ask your GP or practice nurse what help is available in your area and you will be surprised by the variety.

## Orlistat

Over the years I have seen a number of medications come and go in the fight to help people struggling with their weight. Most have been withdrawn because of significant side effects, but one remains. Orlistat is available, without prescription from your pharmacist in half strength (60 mg, three times a day), or on prescription in full strength (120 mg, three times a day). It is licensed for people who are clinically obese, in other words who have a BMI of 30 or more, and who have received at least three months of supervised diet and exercise programmes but without significant weight loss. It can sometimes be given to people with a BMI of 28 or more if they have what we call other obesity-related comorbidities, such as diabetes, heart disease, high blood pressure or sleep apnoea.

Orlistat is a lipase inhibitor. Lipase is an enzyme that helps us to absorb fat from our diet and this drug works by preventing that action. It is vital that the medication is used in conjunction with a low-fat diet. If not, you are likely to experience quite unpleasant fatty diarrhoea and leakage – think of the orange oil left at the bottom of a takeaway curry and that is what might leak from your bottom – so it really is worth sticking to the diet and cutting back on processed food! Orlistat needs to be taken three times a day before meals, and it may help you lose between two and five kilos over a year. Sadly, most patients seem to regain their weight after stopping the drug, although it can take three years to regain the weight lost in 12 months.

## Weight loss surgery

Weight loss surgery, or **bariatric surgery** as it is also called, has become very popular as various celebrities have gone for this option. There is no doubt that it works, but it shouldn't be seen as a panacea. Surgery is a major commitment and, by definition, if you are considering it you must be unhealthily overweight, which has its own implications in terms of anaesthetic risk. Of course, the specialists performing these procedures are very experienced in dealing with larger people, but it is vital that you are well-prepared before going down this route. Below are some of the procedures offered to patients whose weight is compromising their health and who can't seem to get back on track with diet and exercise alone. These are sometimes offered on the NHS, so certainly worth discussing with your doctor.

## Gastric band surgery

Gastric banding is done by keyhole surgery and works by reducing the size of your stomach so that you feel full sooner. It is generally offered to people who are considered to be morbidly obese – that is, those who have a body mass index of over 40, or have a BMI between 30 and 40 and who have already developed other conditions linked to their weight such as diabetes, heart disease or high blood pressure. During the procedure, the surgeon fits an adjustable band around the top of the stomach. He leaves a small opening in the band so that food can pass down to the lower part of the stomach but, by restricting the upper volume, your brain thinks it is full after very small amounts of food. The operation is often done as a day-case procedure (in other words you come in and go home on the same day), or you may need to stay one night. You will than be seen regularly for follow up, where your specialist can inject fluid into the band to tighten it or remove fluid to loosen it depending on how you are getting on. Once the food passes through to the lower stomach, it continues through the rest of the gut and is absorbed normally. Gastric band surgery works because you can't tolerate large amounts of food. You will need to learn to chew your food thoroughly. You should avoid fizzy drinks altogether after this type of surgery, as the bubbles can mean that the band slips. It is not a cure-all – I have met people who have liquidized Mars Bars following this procedure to get their chocolate fix and of course you don't have to do that many times a day to ensure that, small volumes or not, you are getting plenty of calories! One advantage of the gastric band over some of the other weight loss operations you may be offered is that it is entirely reversible and you can have the band removed at any time.

## Gastric sleeve surgery

Gastric sleeve surgery is a more serious procedure than gastric band surgery as it involves having three-quarters of the stomach removed; the remaining part of the stomach then acts as a narrow tube or sleeve, hence the name. It is carried out under general anaesthetic and can be done by keyhole surgery or as an open operation with an incision in your abdomen. It works for two reasons. First, the remaining stomach has a much reduced capacity so you feel full sooner, and second, the part of the stomach that is removed produces some of the hunger hormones that tell your brain you are hungry, so many people describe a reduction in appetite following the procedure and it is common for people to lose weight more quickly than with a gastric band. Unlike the gastric band, this is not a reversible procedure. Once part of the stomach is removed, it cannot be replaced so you need to be absolutely sure this is the right option for you. As this is a more major procedure, you will probably stay in hospital for a few days while you recover.

## Gastric balloon surgery

Gastric balloon surgery is a relatively simple procedure where a small balloon is placed into the stomach using a medical telescope called an **endoscope**. The presence of the balloon feels strange to begin with and some people find they cannot tolerate it and need to have the balloon removed because of nausea and vomiting. As with the band, this is a reversible procedure.

## Gastric bypass surgery

Gastric bypass surgery needs serious consideration; not only is it irreversible, it is a major operation. First, the surgeon creates a smaller stomach using staples and then he or she connects your intestine to this smaller stomach. This means that you have a reduced capacity stomach and, then what you do eat bypasses much of your intestines, where a lot of the nutrients and calories are absorbed. It results in significant weight loss, but you will need professional support to ensure that you don't become deficient in certain nutrients.

# 11

# Metabolic syndrome

The metabolic syndrome is becoming increasingly common in developed countries. Between 20 and 25 per cent of all adults in developed countries currently have metabolic syndrome, and that percentage is likely to increase. It is basically a collection of risk factors for cardiovascular disease, which, it is thought, may be linked in many to **insulin resistance**. Insulin is a hormone that is produced by the pancreas. Its function is to regulate blood sugar levels and keep them within the normal range.

## How is metabolic syndrome diagnosed?

There have been various definitions of the syndrome over the years but, in 2009, the American Heart Association (AHA) and the International Diabetes Federation (IDF) joined forces to come up with a definition that says that if an individual is over 16 years old and has three or more of the following risk factors, then they can be diagnosed with the syndrome.

- *Increased waist circumference* For men, a waist size of above 94 cm (37 inches) is one of the metabolic syndrome risk factors, and for women it's 80 cm (32 inches). People of Asian descent are more at risk of developing metabolic syndrome so for Asian men the limit is 90 cm, and 80 cm for Asian women.
- *BMI greater than 30* This is considered to be clinically obese.
- *Raised triglycerides* Triglyceride levels are checked with a blood test and a level over 1.7 mmol/litre is considered a risk factor. It is also considered a risk factor if drug treatment is needed to keep your levels below this.

- *Reduced HDL cholesterol* HDL cholesterol is the 'good' cholesterol. If levels are less than 1.03 mmol/litre in men or less than 1.29 mmol/litre in women this is considered a risk factor. It is also considered a risk factor if levels are higher than this, but only because you are on treatment.
- *Raised blood pressure* Blood pressure consistently greater than 130/85 is a risk factor, or needing treatment to ensure that blood pressure remains below this level.
- *Raised fasting blood sugar* Fasting blood tests are taken on an empty stomach. If the level is greater than 5.6 mmol/ litre this is a risk factor.

In younger children (6–9 years old) diagnosis is based on waist circumference. When we measure children's waists, we plot the results on a graph using charts which tell us what average children measure. If a child's waist circumference lies on what we call the **90th percentile**, or above, that means that they are in the top 10 per cent of children in terms of waist measurement and this warrants further assessment, particularly if there is a family history of conditions such as metabolic syndrome, type 2 diabetes, heart disease, high blood pressure, high cholesterol or obesity. In children aged 10–15, the diagnosis is made if the waist circumference is on the 90th percentile or higher and there are raised lipids (blood fats), raised blood pressure and a fasting glucose of 5.6 mmol/litre or more.

## Does diagnosing metabolic syndrome matter?

There has been much debate about the significance of diagnosing metabolic syndrome. It was always felt that by making such a diagnosis we could pinpoint those at greater risk of developing type 2 diabetes or heart disease. In fact experts now believe that simply assessing individual risk factors for heart disease is just as, if not more, effective at calculating cardiac risk, and a fasting glucose test alone is probably more useful in predicting those at risk of developing type 2 diabetes. What the diagnosis does do though is to ensure that doctors and nurses can co-ordinate care and address all the health issues that these individuals have.

## What should you do if you have metabolic syndrome?

In a nutshell – read this book and act on the advice! Small but consistent changes to your lifestyle can resolve metabolic syndrome. You should treat this diagnosis as a warning shot across your bow. As I have said before, if you are carrying a lot of extra weight, the idea of reducing your BMI back into the healthy range may just seem such a daunting task that you don't even know where to start. The thing to do is to break this down into achievable targets. This morning, before sitting down to write this, I diagnosed a lady with metabolic syndrome. She fits the AHA/IDF metabolic syndrome criteria, and, in fact, has five of the six risk factors. She wants to help herself, but was totally overwhelmed by the prospect of having to lose several stone. When we looked at her parameters in detail her waist circumference, BMI, triglycerides, HDL cholesterol and blood pressure were all outside normal limits – but only just. She undoubtedly has metabolic syndrome and, of course, she should aim for a healthy BMI of between 18.5 and 25 but, in fact, if she lost just 10 per cent of her body weight most of those measurements would come down enough to mean she would no longer be diagnosed with metabolic syndrome. And even if she cannot achieve a normal BMI, she can make a huge difference to the risks to her health in the future.

## Are there medicines for metabolic syndrome?

The AHA doesn't recommend the use of drugs solely to treat metabolic syndrome, but the diabetic drug metformin is sometimes used, particularly in women with metabolic syndrome and polycystic ovaries. This is what we call pre-scribing **off label**. This is when doctors prescribe drugs that are licensed for a different use, but are thought to be helpful for an alternative condition. The doctor should be familiar with the use of that particular drug and should explain to you that he is prescribing off label. Your doctor may also discuss other drugs depending on the results of your tests. He or she may, for example, suggest you take a statin to reduce cholesterol, medication to reduce your blood pressure or anti-diabetic drugs. If you address your weight problems these drugs may not be needed in the long term. As I have said, as your weight drops, your measurements will improve and you may no longer need prescription medication. One word of caution though – don't ever take that into your own hands. It is vital that you discuss with your doctor whether or not you can stop a prescription medicine as some need to be discontinued slowly.

# 12

# Diabetes

In this chapter when I talk about diabetes, I'm referring to diabetes mellitus. Diabetes insipidus is a different condition where you have problems controlling the balance of water in your body. As with diabetes mellitus, it can make you excessively thirsty, but it is not linked to being overweight or obese. It is due to a problem either in the brain or in the kidneys. There are two types of diabetes mellitus. This chapter will deal with type 2 which is by far the more common type, accounting for 90 to 95 per cent of all adult diabetics. Type 1 diabetes is not linked to weight. It is a condition where your body develops antibodies to the beta cells in your pancreas. These are the cells that produce insulin and very quickly your insulin levels drop. Type 1 diabetes is treated with insulin from diagnosis.

## Type 2 diabetes

Type 2 diabetes used to also be called **adult-onset**, or **maturity-onset**, diabetes because it was seen in older people generally over 40. These names have now been dropped because that is no longer the case. Type 2 diabetes is linked to being overweight and, because we are becoming bigger as a nation, and lots of young people are now clinically obese, we are seeing type 2 diabetes in young adults and even in children. Unlike type 1 diabetes, type 2 diabetes develops slowly. If it is picked up early, then it can often be managed with diet alone, but if left untreated will need prescription medication. Ultimately, some type 2 diabetics will need insulin by injection. Type 2 diabetes develops because either you have become resistant to the effects of insulin, so normal insulin levels just aren't enough to keep your blood sugar under control, or your body doesn't make enough insulin. In some cases it can be a mixture of both.

## Who gets type 2 diabetes?

More people than you think! It is estimated that in the UK alone, there are 750,000 people walking around, getting on with their day to day lives, who have diabetes and have no idea. Because the symptoms can be vague, and come on so insidiously, it is perfectly possible to have the condition and not be aware that you are unwell. Risk factors for type 2 diabetes include:

- *Weight* Being clinically overweight (BMI 25–30) or clinically obese (BMI >30) significantly increases your risk and most type 2 diabetics are overweight.
- *Waist circumference* Women with waist circumferences of greater than 80 cm (31.5 inches) and greater than 94 cm (37 inches) for men; or 90 cm (35.5 inches) if you are an Asian or Afro–Caribbean male.
- *Ethnicity* Type 2 diabetes is about five times more common in people of Asian and Afro–Caribbean descent.
- *Family history* If your mother, father, brother, sister or child has diabetes,you are more likely to develop the condition.
- *Impaired glucose tolerance* If it is found, on routine testing, that you have a slightly raised glucose level which is not high enough to make a diagnosis of diabetes but is higher than normal, you will be asked to have what is called a **glucose tolerance test**. This involves having nothing to eat or drink for 8 or 12 hours. You will have a blood test, which is referred to as the 'fasting sample'. You will then be given a sugary drink containing a known amount of glucose and blood samples are taken again at given intervals to see how your body manages that known amount

of sugar. If your body struggles to get your blood sugar level back to the normal range then this is called **impaired glucose tolerance** and puts you at increased risk of developing type 2 diabetes.

- *Pregnancy* If you have impaired glucose tolerance or become diabetic during pregnancy this usually resolves after the baby is born, but it does increase your risk of developing type 2 diabetes later in life.

## How is type 2 diabetes diagnosed?

The symptoms of type 2 diabetes are vague and come on slowly. You may experience lethargy and increased thirst. You may find that you are passing urine more frequently and may have recurrent infections, such as thrush, but because these symptoms develop slowly, over many months, a lot of people don't really notice so most cases of type 2 diabetes are picked up after routine health checks. In the first instance your doctor may notice there is sugar in your urine, which is picked up on urine dipstick testing. If this is found you will be asked to have a blood test, usually on a fasting sample. That means having nothing to eat or drink for several hours (usually about eight hours) before your blood test. **Fasting blood sugar** levels should be between 3.6 mmol/litre and 6.1 mmol/litre. If fasting sugar levels are higher than 7 mmol/litre, or if a what we call a **random glucose level,** i.e. one taken at any time of the day, is greater than 11.1 mmol/litre, this is diagnostic of diabetes. If an individual has no symptoms but the abnormality is picked up on routine testing, then we repeat the tests to confirm the diagnosis but one test is enough for diagnosis if a person has symptoms of type 2 diabetes. We also use another blood test called the **HbA1c** test. This is a measure of what has been happening to blood sugar levels over recent weeks. If it's greater than 6.5 per cent, this is diagnostic of diabetes.

It is also a test that is used to monitor how well diabetes is controlled following diagnosis.

## How is type 2 diabetes managed?

In the first instance you will probably be asked to have an appointment with the practice nurse to talk through what you can do to change your diet and lifestyle. For some, lifestyle changes alone may be all that is needed, but it is important that you know exactly what you can and can't eat. It may feel daunting at first but, to be honest, much of what I have already said in this book will be relevant to you. While you are waiting for that appointment, try to keep a food diary so that the nurse (and you!) can see where you are going wrong and give you some tips on how you manage your eating habits in the future. You will need to adopt a low-fat, low-salt and low-sugar diet. Low fat, because managing your weight is crucial, low salt because diabetics are prone to high blood pressure and kidney problems, and low sugar because, by definition, diabetics have difficulty handling and processing sugar; of course, low sugar will help keep your weight under control too. As a rough guide, your diet should look like this:

- total fat less than 35 per cent of total calorie intake;
- trans fats and saturated fats should constitute less than 33 per cent of total fat intake;
- total carbohydrates should make up 40–60 per cent of your total calorie intake.

It's tough but you can reduce your fat intake by limiting fried or processed foods and high-fat snacks, such as crisps, cake and biscuits; you will also need to be careful with fizzy drinks, squashes and cordials and limit cakes and biscuits. You should choose foods with a **low glycaemic index**, which means foods that produce less of a peak in blood sugar levels. So, for example, the blood sugar peak seen after eating pasta is much lower than that after eating chips because pasta has a lower glycaemic index than potato.

Not everyone with type 2 diabetes is overweight, but the majority are and tackling this will be a priority for you. It is likely to be a long haul but even modest weight loss can make a real difference. Depending on the blood results, your GP and nurse may suggest that you look at lifestyle changes alone for a few months. If they can see your HbA1c returning to normal as a result of these changes then you may not need to do anything further.

### What if my blood tests remain abnormal?

If your blood tests remain abnormal despite making changes to your lifestyle, your doctor will prescribe medication to help bring your blood sugar levels under control. It is important that you persevere with your lifestyle changes, as even if you need medication now, as you continue to bring your weight down and improve your fitness you may find that you will be able to come off your medication. Although, as I have said before, don't ever be tempted to try this without the help of your doctor.

There are several types of tablets used to keep blood sugar levels under control.

**Metformin** The drug metformin is a biguanide. It works by enhancing the use of available glucose. It is the first drug we use in type 2 diabetes that is associated with weight issues and, since most, although not all, type 2 diabetics are overweight, this is the first drug of choice. It improves sensitivity to insulin and may help with weight loss.

**Nateglinide and repaglinide** These drugs stimulate the release of insulin. They work very quickly after being taken, but they don't last for long so they are taken immediately before eating. Nateglinide is only licensed to be used in conjunction with metformin, but repaglinide can be used on its own in type 2 diabetics who are not overweight or who cannot tolerate metformin. It causes weight gain.

**Sulfonylureas**  These drugs work by enhancing insulin secretion, so by definition they are only useful if the pancreas is capable of producing some insulin. There are different sulfonylureas and which one you are prescribed will depend on your individual circumstances. They have different lengths of action: that is, depending on which type you have, each dose you take works for a different length of time – some of the more long-acting types may put you at risk of becoming hypoglycaemic, meaning that your blood sugar falls too low. This can be a medical emergency, so your doctor will fine tune which particular sulfonylurea is best for you. The sulfonylureas include glibenclamide, gliclazide, glimepiride, glipizide and tolbutamide. Sadly, they tend to cause weight gain.

**Pioglitazone**  This drug works by reducing insulin resistance. It can be used on its own or alongside other medicines but it must be used with care. It has been shown to increase the risk of heart failure when combined with insulin, so shouldn't be used in anyone with known heart failure, and all patients who take this drug need to be closely monitored.

**Gliptins**  These drugs increase insulin secretion and reduce glucagon secretion. Glucagon is another pancreatic hormone which works to raise blood sugar levels when they start to fall. Gliptins can be used on their own or in conjunction with other medicines. They include saxagliptin, sitagliptin and vildagliptin.

**Acarbose**  This drug delays the digestion and absorption of carbohydrate and sugar from the gut. It is generally reserved for those patients who cannot tolerate other anti-diabetic medication.

## What if tablets can't control my type 2 diabetes?

If you have tried lifestyle changes and, despite adding in tablets, your sugar levels and HbA1c levels remain abnormal your doctor will suggest you try injection therapy. There are two main types of injection therapy.

- *Insulin* Insulin injections can be given as individual injections and there are many different types. Some are short acting, meaning their effect doesn't last long, some have intermediate action and some are long acting. You may well need a combination of different types. Insulin can also be given via a pump which means fewer injections. If you are injecting regularly you will be advised to rotate your injection sites as repeated injections at the same site will be uncomfortable and can cause changes in the underlying fatty tissue. This is called **lipodystrophy** and looks like dimples and lumps under the skin.
- *Exenatide and liraglutide* These drugs increase insulin secretion, reduce glucagon secretion and delay gastric emptying so that there is a slower delivery of food to the small intestine where the sugar is absorbed.

### Will I need other medication?

If you are diabetic your risk of developing high blood pressure, high cholesterol and heart disease among other things, increases. Your doctor will want to monitor you for these problems and will advise on whether you need medication. The good news through all of this, though, is that if you persevere with your lifestyle changes you could potentially, under the supervision of your medical team, come off all the medicines. That is quite some incentive!

## How will my diabetes be monitored?

You will need regular review at your GP surgery and maybe also at the hospital. You will need blood tests to check your glucose levels and your HbA1c and you will also need cholesterol blood tests, and tests to check your kidney function. You will have your eyes checked every year as diabetes can affect your vision and you will have regular blood pressure checks, and checks on your sensation and your feet. It is important that whenever you have an appointment that you leave knowing when the next one will be, and whether it is down to you to make a note of when to go back, or whether you will be informed when it is nearer the appointment date.

## Why is it so important to control my sugar level when I don't feel unwell?

You may feel totally well with higher than normal blood sugar levels but persistently high glucose levels in the blood damage the blood vessels, the body's organs and the nerves. In real terms, this means that if you ignore your condition you are at significant risk of some serious health issues in the future. These include:

### Heart disease and stroke

Diabetics are up to five times more likely to have a heart attack or stroke because they are more likely to develop furring of the arteries. This could present as angina where, classically, you experience a crushing central chest pain on exertion or after eating a meal. The pain sometimes radiates to the jaw or the left arm and may be associated with shortness of breath and nausea. Pain like this should never be ignored and needs urgent medical attention. If the pain persists, it could indicate that you are having a heart attack and need to call an ambulance immediately. A stroke may present as slurring of your speech, drooping on one side of your face or weakness in your arms and or legs.

## High blood pressure

Diabetics are more prone to high blood pressure as the arteries become narrower. It is completely normal for your blood pressure to go up when you are anxious, in pain or exercising, but if blood pressure is consistently raised this puts a strain on your heart. I liken it to driving a car. If you put your foot on the throttle occasionally to accelerate past an obstacle, your car will cope fine, but if you drive around constantly with your foot on the floor, it won't be long before the engine starts to struggle. If your arteries are narrowed and the same volume of blood needs to be pumped around by your heart then it stands to reason that your heart is having to work harder to force the blood around your body.

## High cholesterol

Diabetics are prone to high cholesterol and if you are a diabetic, your doctor will be keen to keep your cholesterol levels lower than if you were a non-diabetic.

## Visual problems

Poor diabetic control can make the small blood vessels that supply the retina (the light-sensitive membrane at the back of the eye) to become blocked or leaky and if left unchecked this can lead to blindness. This is called **diabetic retinopathy**. The human brain and eye compensate very well for gradual loss of vision so you may not be aware that you are developing a problem until it is too late. If you are known to be diabetic and are registered with an NHS GP, you will automatically be called every year for a special eye test. If changes are caught early they can often be treated with laser therapy to prevent things getting worse.

### Kidney disease

If the blood supply to your kidneys is affected by diabetes then your kidneys can't work as well. If left unchecked this can lead to kidney failure and would mean you need dialysis or possibly a kidney transplant. Keeping your blood sugar levels well controlled can help prevent this.

### Nerve damage

It's not just the large blood vessels that are damaged by high sugar levels. The very tiny vessels that supply your nerves can also be affected and this can lead to a burning sensation known as **neuralgia**. It can also lead to numbness, which means you may not feel things normally. If I have a small stone in my shoe, it causes me pain and I will take my shoe off and remove the stone. If your nerves have been damaged by diabetes, you may not be aware of that stone and so could potentially walk around on it all day. This could lead to an ulcer forming and, because of the circulatory problems common in diabetes, this may be very difficult to heal. If the nerves to the gut are affected, it can cause big problems with diarrhoea or constipation.

### Foot problems

The combination of nerve damage and poor circulation make diabetics more prone to ulceration and infection. This is one reason why diabetics are entitled to free podiatry on the NHS and, if you are diabetic, it is well worth getting your feet checked regularly. If you struggle with nail cutting, for example, a podiatrist or chiropodist can do this for you to ensure that you don't cut your skin.

### Sexual problems

Diabetic men are more likely to develop erectile dysfunction due to nerve and blood vessel damage. Even if you think this isn't a problem for you, you should mention it your doctor as it could be an indication that you have other circulatory problems that need checking out.

## Stillbirth and miscarriage

Diabetic women who become pregnant tend to have bigger babies or are more likely to miscarry or have a stillbirth. Most antenatal care today is provided by midwives in the community but, if you are diabetic, then you are likely to be looked after in hospital to minimize any risks.

## Travelling with diabetes

Diabetes shouldn't mean you can't travel, but it will mean that you have to plan ahead. Delays to your journey could be an issue for you and, as mealtimes may be a little unpredictable, it is worth always carrying carbohydrate snacks with you so that you have control over when you eat. If you are going away for any length of time take a copy of your prescription with you so that you can tell a doctor exactly what you are on in case you should lose your medication. If you are flying, keep your medication with you in hand luggage so, should there be any delays, you have it with you; if you need to use needles, ask your doctor for a letter explaining why you need to carry them with you to avoid any problems with airport security.

## Can I drive with diabetes?

If you are a driver with a group 1 licence (cars and motorbikes), you must tell the DVLA if you are taking insulin for more than three months and they will arrange for you to have your licence reviewed every one, two or three years. If you are a group 2 driver (buses or lorries), you must inform the DVLA if you are on any medication, and that includes tablets. They will require you to attend for an independent medical check every year where you will be asked to provide details of regular blood sugar checks on a meter.

# Index